Medical Residency Interview Questions

Answers & Insights

Notes & Key Points

OLAREWAJU OLADIPO, MD

Book

D1285980

FOREWORD

Every Match season bears its unique sets of challenges, not only for the applicants, but for all those who are charged with ensuring that the process runs smoothly. While several of the challenges are simple replica of prior seasons, some outright new challenges sometime surface. This book pertains to one critical aspect of this whole process – the interview. The interview process remains one aspect of the whole residency application process upon which the final decision regarding candidate selection is made. In clear terms, it means that the performance of an applicant during the interview process cannot be underestimated in terms of what role it plays in the selection process.

In many instances, due to the mismatch between the number of available training positions and the overall count of applicants, a significant proportion of applicants do not make it to the interview stage. Nevertheless, it is prudent that every applicant prepare adequately for the interview process, irrespective of their score profile or potential for selectivity. Without any disregard to the importance of the other aspects of a resident's application package, the interview is what clinches the deal for many. As such, it is prudent that every applicant prepare adequately for the opportunity of an interview.

While the important aspects of a residency application package include having great scores, obtaining strong letters of references, and possessing an excellent resume and a well-crafted personal statement, the interview is one aspect that cannot be ignored; not even for the most desirable of applicants. This book is an effort to support the applicant in their preparatory effort.

Contrary to what may be obtainable with other texts on this subject, this book was written to offer the reader various insights on the different dimensions that a particular question may take, and to reinforce the fact that a formulaic response may not be adequate in all instances that an applicant is presented with such a question.

As you proceed to read this book, you will observe that at every opportunity, great effort is devoted to stimulating the reader to develop a structure that fits their personal story, and to approach each question with that in mind, and not to lose the opportunity that a question may offer in terms of having a memorable conversation. It will also become clearer to the reader that the same amount of effort was implemented in steering the conversation away from a rehearsed response tactic. In using this approach, the reader is encouraged to view the interview process as a unique opportunity to connect with the interviewer.

The value of this book is inherent in the fact that the author was able to tap into an enormous wealth of experience, one that was acquired over the course of several years in the course of mentoring and coaching international medical graduates applying for residency training opportunities. While this book was inspired by the privilege of engaging with this unique group of applicants, a good proportion of who may not be well equipped for the various nuances of local interview practices, it is an invaluable tool for anyone going through the interview process. Having successfully prepared hundreds of applicants for the yearly Match, one observation that stands out is the fact that having a great interview is never an accident, but one that is rooted in deliberate preparation, ordered practice, and a determination to improve on the current level of performance.

The brevity of this book was intentional, with each page packed with the essentials that are needed for the reader to succeed at any interview. It is my hope that the reader finds the wisdom of this book useful, and discovers ways to apply the knowledge as the interview season approaches.

ACKNOWLEDGEMENT

This book is dedicated to the all those who have and continue to support the collective effort of KAINJI in mentoring medical professionals pursuing career advancement opportunities. To learn more about our mission, visit www.kainji.org

♣ 1. What do you hope to gain from our residency program?

Insight

This question is a direct variant of what a particular training program means to you. It may come in other direct forms, as in **'*what can our program offer you?*'**, **'what does this program mean to you?'** , **'why did you choose this program?', 'what are you looking for in our program', 'what makes this program special to you?'**, or **'why this program?'** While the question itself may seem like an easy opportunity to focus on the obvious, and state the common reasons why one would choose a great program, it is advisable to think deeply about you as a person, and consider your immediate goals, as well as your future aspirations. Paramount among the reasons that apply to you will be those that tie into your short term goal, but it is an opportunity to share how relevant the reasons are to your future plans.

Knowing that many applicants will present a similar set of generic points, some of which may border on mediocrity, there is a real opportunity for you to stand out as an applicant in this instance. It is generally assumed that every applicant is well prepared for this question, whatever format it may take. Nevertheless, many applicants limit themselves to stating the obvious, such as the desire to obtain an excellent training, gain essential clinical skills, and have the opportunity to connect with great mentors. Having one or two points that is peculiar to your situation or your application will demonstrate your seriousness about the program.

A bit of prior research will definitely serve you well in this instance, as it may yield unique observations that may enable you to readily connect with the interviewer. Rather than limit yourself to the generic list of what a program can offer you, it is advisable to structure your responses away from the formal style, but in the direction of a more realistic conversation.

Answer

Apart from the obvious reasons why anyone would choose to apply to **UCH,** such as its record of training **excellent physicians**, many of who have gone on to make significant contributions in the field, and its reputation for having a great faculty, I decided to apply to this program for two main reasons.

One relates to my personal circumstance. I have elderly immigrant parents who live about an hour away from where this program is located. It will mean so much to me if I am able to undergo residency training at a location that is not too distant from them. As their only adult child, they often rely on me for their medical appointment and other routine errands.

The other pertains to my interest in Addiction Medicine. I am familiar with the work of **Dr. Onyeaka**, her numerous publications and her involvement with serving the local community. I consider having an exposure to such a community and learning from her and colleagues will be one special opportunity.

Notes

It is important to note the highlighted texts in the preceding pages. The following comments further explains their significance.

- *'UCH'*, the name of the training program brings a level of authenticity to the conversation. This is particularly important to the interviewer who may assume that you have several other interviews to attend.

- *'excellent physicians'*, is not specific enough as a general comment, and it may be important to attach one or two names to this particular line. The names does not necessarily need to be some highly acclaimed physician, and could be one or two residents that passed through the training program in recent years; such individuals may undergoing fellowship training, or may have completed training and are in clinical practice.

- *'Dr. Onyeaka'*, as a reference point, may become a subject of further conversation, especially if you claim to be familiar with her work in a particular field and a few of her publications. It is therefore advisable that you only make such a reference only if you are confident with handling the follow-up question that may ensue.

Key Points

In preparing for the various forms that this question may take, the key point is to identify the obvious reasons, state a few if time permits, but to use the opportunity to address one or two reasons that resonate with your situation. It in this wisdom that you are able to turn an ordinary interview to a memorable encounter.

Worksheet

♣ 2. What are your long term goals?

Insight

One question that I often get asked by applicants is the clear definition of 'long term goals.' Rather than focus on a precise definition centered on a specific calendar, be creative in owning the definition in how it relates to attaining a set goal. While an older graduate, in my early forties, long term goals have a different meaning, the same may not be the case with a twenty-nine year applicant. Taking such an approach to dealing with this question simplifies the way you choose to answer the question.

Since this interview relates to the career of the individual as a resident and a future career as a physician, it is important that you stay on point in the way you respond to the question. By doing so, you avoid any undesirable attention that may limit your opportunities for getting into your choice of residency position. Ii is not the moment to reveal your intention to become a medical expert on a TV soap series, or wanting to use the opportunity to pursue a career in acting.

Long term goals, from the standpoint of the interviewer often relate to the plans for the future in terms of clinical practice, research, academics, community work or medical outreach. While I consider this question a favorable one from the point of the interviewee, I see it as non-consequential in a sense, especially as it relates to an applicant's suitability for the training program. Unlike short term goals that pertain to the training years and the immediate period following those years, long term goals can be as vague and as esoteric as one decides to make it. Having said that, it makes sense to be specific in your overall presentation, but instead, you should find ways to connect the opportunity that you are currently seeking with those plans that you consider as future goals.

Lastly, one should not forget the different forms that this question may take. Examples of such include **'*where do you see yourself a decade from now?*'** or **'what do you see yourself doing ten years from now?' or 'how does this opportunity of a residency position tie into your long term goals?'**

In all these questions, except for the last, the format is fairly direct. In the last question, the applicant is present with a 'combination of two questions - one directed at getting an answer to what you hope to gain from the opportunity you are pursuing, and the other directed at finding out what your long term goals are.

This particular set of questions may eliminate the temporal nature of the question, in which case it could simply be presented as a question about your goals, both short term and long term. When such is the case, the approach to the question will similar, but with emphasis on both your short term and long term goals, whatever time frame you decide to use to classify them.

Answer

In responding to this question, I would like to define 'long term' as that period starting after I have completed my residency training in Radiology, and at least experienced two to three years of clinical practice, preferably in an academic setting. That makes it roughly **'seven to ten years'** from now. At that point, I plan to transition to a private practice setting, while at the same time, take up a part-time teaching appointment at the medical school.

In fact, since my medical school years, I have had a deep interest in mentoring as well as teaching, especially in the medical field and working with young women pursuing careers in Radiology.

I would also like to point out that one of the reason that I applied to your program is its record of successfully guiding women in the profession into positions of leadership. I am particularly familiar with the career trajectory of **'Dr. Ogbonda'**, and how she has advanced in the field of Radiology. I believe that over time, I am able to build a long term relationship with the medical school, such that I can continue to play a role in such a capacity.

Notes

It is important to note the highlighted texts in the preceding pages. The following comments further explains their significance.

- **'seven to ten years'**, is the definition that was utilized in addressing the question of long term goal, in this instance. Rather than the interviewee boxing himself or herself into a fixed time period, by identifying specific career milestones, he or she is able to set realistic expectations that targets is better comprehended by the interviewer.

- *Specificity*, with respect to what your long term goals are will limit the vagueness that is often encountered in the way applicants tackle this particular question. It also helps to break it into specifics that are more realistic in the eyes of the interviewer. In the example of the response generated to this question, the specifics include securing work in private practice, taking up partial teaching responsibilities and the mentoring of young women in the professions.

- **'Dr. Ogbonda',** is another example of healthy name-dropping, that may help to further explain to the interviewer that you have done your homework, and have good reasons for applying to their training program.

Key Points

Now that you are more familiar with the various forms that this question might take, it makes sense to draw up your future goals across a variety of time frames. One recommendation is to complete a career plan chart for three periods – five-year post residency, ten-year post residency, and fifteen-year post residency. That way, you will always be prepared to tackle whatever form the question takes, and you are well placed to communicate the facts to your interviewer.

Worksheet

♣ 3. What do you consider to be your strengths?

Insight

In the many interview practice sessions that I have participated in, this particular question comes up often, yet the feedback from scores of applicants who have attended interviews over the past years revealed that the question is not as common as we make it seem. In my role, reviewing personal statements written by applicants who are planning to apply for residency positions, an applicant's personal statement tends to do a better job dealing with this aspect of a candidate. In fact, one can readily carve out a short paragraph to address this particular aspect of the application.

In every sense, the so-called strengths overlap with the personality traits that are critical for success in our day-to-day relationship, and tend to be addressed during interview from that angle. It so happens that the desirable qualities expected of any applicant fall under the same umbrella – hardworking, consistent, considerate, amiable, determined, flexible, motivated, determined, resourceful, creative, and so on and so forth. That been the case, simply reiterating these attributes may not offer an applicant any opportunity to outshine fellow applicants, who are very likely to state the same qualities.

While such an approach is not totally flawed, its impact is less impressive and may not yield much of an advantage when the number of applicants competing for a chosen position far outstrips the available opportunities. One of the recommended ways to personalize the response is to associate the chosen attributes to an experience that is unique to you as an applicant. This is where storytelling becomes a useful tool, and provided there is adequate time on the interview schedule to demonstrate such a talent, you can choose this route to highlight some of your strengths. In the next section, a mixed approach will be implemented in addressing the question.

Answer

In addition to the typical strengths that defines a desirable residency applicant, such as great work ethics, ability to cope with the demand of work, consistency of performance, and excellent communication skills, I recently had the opportunity to demonstrate one of my attributes during a work situation.

This actually happened about two months ago, while I was undergoing a rotation at suburban hospital. After an overnight work schedule, a professional colleague failed to turn up to work on schedule; I mean two hours later than the starting time. While a few of my fellow colleagues were upset with the disruption in the workflow for the day, I was more concerned for the wellbeing of the work colleague. Rather than go home immediately after handing over, I self-nominated to continue with his allocated work duties pending when he reports for work later that morning.

When the colleague finally presented for work, we learned that his apartment was burgled the night before, and he had lost the use of his car as well as his phone. It was one memorable moments when I had the opportunity to demonstrate exercise patience, show a degree of maturity, and show the willingness to make a sacrifice on behalf of someone else.

Notes

It is important to note the highlighted texts in the preceding pages. The following comments further explains their significance.

'the list', approach was utilized as a starting point in answering this question, enabling the applicant to state some positive attributes consistent with his strength, "great work ethics, ability to cope with the demand of work, consistency of performance, and excellent communication skills…." This style, at least offers an opportunity to reveal s=the salient ones, while to explore the option of storytelling.

'storytelling', may not always be feasible, depending on the format of the interview, preference of the interviewer and the allocation of time.

'a healthy dose of narcissism', is unavoidable in this instance, as a formal interview is one of the few moments when you will be called upon to talk about yourself, and present the desirable attributes that make you worthy of the offer of a coveted position. The tricky point when it comes to dealing with this question is to balance the conversation such that one is able to convey the necessary information without sounding boastful.

Key Points

In preparing for a question like this, you have to become comfortable with the idea of selling yourself, even if that is not your usual nature. This is often the case with individuals coming from a culture where humility is sometimes exercised to the extreme. In guiding residency applicants through this particular question, the recommendation to have this question in a written form such that you can readily adopt it for use as the interview situation demands. With respect to the storytelling component, that is not always going to be possible in all instances, and rather than concoct a story that is inauthentic, it is better to stick to the 'list' in addressing the question.

Worksheet

♣ 4. Tell me how you handled a difficult situation. How did you manage?

Insight

This particular question, while it regularly features during interview sessions, needs to be handled with care. In the open-ended format that is utilized in this example, the interviewer is less clear about the premise of the so-called, 'difficult situation', and the applicant is left with the task of choosing the direction of the conversation. In a way, it could be a blessing in a way as you are free to choose which way to proceed. Generally speaking, since this question is being presented in the setting of an interview for a residency position, It may be prudent on your part to confirm with the interviewer whether the answer should be limited to a work situation, or life in general. That way, you are not unfairly penalized for running off in a wrong direction.

For the purpose of practicing for such a question, it is not a bad idea if you actually prepare to answer such a question from the standpoint of a professional event as in clinical work, research, or study to do with the profession, as well as in a domestic setting that has to do with the business of living. Using such an approach in your preparatory effort means that one is not surprised by the interviewer.

As it is the case with the other questions that are addressed in this book, it is important to remember that there are a few variants to this question, from the more specific as in a stipulated case scenario to the broad, open-ended form, like the one addressed in this section. Sample variants include, **'how did you resolve a difficult situation at work?'**, **'have you encountered any challenging situation that you had to address?'**, **'tell me of a disappointing incident that you had to cope with'**, or **'tell me of a difficult clinical experience you once encountered in your practice of medicine'**. In all these questions, the interviewer is interested in the challenging situation as much as in how you managed to resolve the situation. In the right setting, this question, or any of its variant offers you the opportunity to weave into the story a number of information that takes more than one question to obtain from an applicant. Not only are you able to talk about yourself, it's a window to shed some light on your past or current work as it relates to the experience you choose to share.

Answer

In answering this question, I will relate an challenging situation that happened recently in my current position as a junior medical officer. Even though it was social and clinical in nature, it was my first experience of dealing with such a situation. It also required that use a combination of life skills and clinical acumen to establish a true diagnosis as well as take necessary steps.

The situation pertains to my encounter with a patient of domestic violence and how the patient had concealed the fact from me on two separate prior occasions. Even though I had my suspicion during the prior encounters, the patient vehemently denied that being the case, and I had treated the bruises on her left thigh as the result of separate accidental falls. It was at the time of the third encounter, when I point blank accused the patient of lying that the incident happened. Not only did she deny that my judgement was wrong, she threatened to report me to the hospital administration. I was now faced with a dilemma, between standing my ground or ignoring the situation until it gets out of hand. Rather than simply capitulate, I thought of an alternative strategy to deal with the situation. During that same appointment, she agreed to continue treatment under the care of a senior colleague in the practice; In a subsequent visit, a few days later, she acquiesced and acknowledged the issue of domestic violence by her husband.

In de-escalating the situation, I not only avoided a confrontation with the patient, I displayed a genuine concern for the welfare of the patient by providing an easy alternative. It was such quick thinking that eventually resulted in her decision to acknowledged the problem at hand, agree to the recommendation for proper intervention. Not too long after that incident, during one of her subsequent appointment at the clinic, she stopped by at my office, and offered an apology for her behavior during our last encounter, and for her unruly behavior.

Notes

It is obvious that my approach to the question took the route of an incident pertaining to my practice of medicine. It felt natural and comforting, as I did not want to narrate an event related to a personal o domestic situation to an interviewer that I have never met before. This approach also meant that I gave myself the chance for subsequent questions by the interviewer aligns with my clinical experience.

'conflict negotiation', a useful skill applicable to both work and life situations was one quality that this story revealed about the applicant. It not only reveal a little bit of the applicants personality in terms of temperament, it also showed the astuteness of the applicant with respect to problem-solving.

'do no harm', a mantra often expressed in the practice of medicine was exercised in the applicant's interaction with the patient. While the patient's reaction may have resulted in a summary discharge from the clinic, her physician was more concerned with getting to the root of the situation, thereby offering her the choice of another physician.

'reconciliation', an outcome that was the outcome of the previously noted characteristics of this story. It is not often in the course of clinical practice that a patient walks into one's office to tender an unsolicited apology.

Key Points

In this one question, the interviewee readily displayed several qualities that truly tells of her personality, professional attitude and her emotional maturity. Preparing a response using the event of a clinical or work setting is a preferred option, and avoids an unnecessary diversion into an applicant's personal life.

It is generally a good idea to write out a draft of one or two scenarios, like the one narrated in this section, well-tailored to your professional experience, and showing some qualities you would like the interviewer to be aware of. I believe there are ample opportunities to recount one or two real life stories in your work experience, as the life of a physician meant that you are constantly presented with difficult situations in the course of caring for patients.

Worksheet

♣ 5. Tell me of one experience of having to deal with failure, and how dealt with it.

Insight

There are certain questions that offer the opportunity to connect with the interviewer; this question is one of them. Since the subject of failure is something that many physicians would have had to grapple with in the course of their careers, it is quite likely that an interviewer would be able to relate to your version of a story that deals with this question.

My take on this question is to make it simple and keep it to an event that relates to your career journey. While it is easy to readily settle for an experience to do with failing a professional examination, or one to do with an unfavorable outcome with respect to the care of a patient, it is recommended that the applicant take the time to search for an event that offers the chance to stand out among fellow interviewees. This particular question is not usually one of those that you decide on a suitable response at the time of the interview. Since it is agreed that you have had the time to prepare for the interview, it is expected that you have at least one, or more drafts of an experience that enables you to readily tackle this question.

Like many of the other questions featured in this book, it is inevitable that you would have to master the process of storytelling as part of your preparation for the interview season. Both the experience of failure and your approach to handling the disappointment become your ticket to securing a memorable encounter. On many occasions, an applicant's response to this question became critical during the selection process, and resulting in the decision by the selection committee to choose one applicant over the others.

Answer

Permit me to take you to a time well before I got into medical school. As an orphan, charting my path through medical school was a lesson in perseverance and one that I would like to share in answering this question. In was at the end of my high school year and having gained the offer of an admission for undergraduate studies in Microbiology, I had applied for a scholarship to cover both the tuition and my tuition expenses. After a preliminary round of selection where over two hundred applicants were whittled down to a dozen, I was confident that I would win one of the five of the offered scholarship. For some reason, having put my heart into the preparing for the essay and interview to claim one of the prizes, I was very confident in my ability and of the eventual outcome.

It was therefore devastating when I discovered that I was not one of the successful applicants. You could imagine, and at the time, aged seventeen, it seemed like my world had crashed. Well, after sobbing for a few days, and my friends have done their share of consoling me, I had to try my best to move forward. It was not particularly easy, and I don't think I fully remember how I survived. But, somehow, I did. It took a combination of prayer, sheer determination, and a decision to take one day at a time. Miraculously, I somehow made it through college.

It is interesting to know that the experience of that disappointment became my winning ticket when it was time to apply for a scholarship to attend medical school. One of the essay questions was a narrative on a personal experience of failure and how I managed to cope with it. That later success taught me to take my failure in stride, to carry on despite the odds, and to use the pain of the experience as a fuel for travel toward my final destination.

Notes

As you would notice, it is not uncommon for anyone to share an experience of failure without generating one form of emotion or the other. On many occasions, I have heard feedback from interviewers when an interviewer was brought to tears with an applicant's story. Not a particularly comfortable position to find oneself as an applicant, to be labelled as that applicant that made the interviewer cry. Often, such occurrences are totally beyond our control, as the same experience shared with other interviewers may not show any connection whatsoever.

While it should never be your intention as an applicant to trigger such an emotion, the authenticity of your storyteller is what dictates how the listener reacts to your narrative. In fact, the story narrated by the applicant does not necessarily have to be gloomy to resonate with an interviewer.

'authenticity, is the secret to doing this question the full justice it deserves. This means that you should be true to yourself, and feel free to express the way you felt at the time in question.

'no history of failure', is not an excuse to recuse yourself from the question. While you may use the opportunity to reveal you overall fortune with your journey so far in life, I am sure you can remember some not so trivial event in your life. Such events may include losing a tracking competition, an unsuccessful bid for a leadership position at college, or even failing to win a medal a your high school tracking event or chess competition. The key is not to let such a question go to waste.

'coping with failure', is not unique to one individual, and as such may not particularly identify you from a pool of qualified applicants. While it makes sense to highlight the steps that you took to create an opportunity at a future date, be natural in your presentation, and do not dwell too much on this aspect such that the story itself loses its relevance. It is also worth noting that even when the question did not specifically ask you to narrate how you coped with failure or disappointment, that you try to include it in your response.

Key Points

It is important that you have a version of an experience that fits into whatever version this question takes. In my experience dealing with applicants undergoing interviews for residency training positions, this question tends to feature more often than other somewhat over-rated questions.

This particular question is also very important from the perspective of a physician, knowing that the reality of medical practice dictates that you will face disappointments, and may have to prepare yourself to better handle failures when they do manifest.

Lastly, as we have done in prior sections of this book, the variants of this question include, **'tell me about how you handled a personal disappointment'**, **'tell about an experience of failure in your journey so far'**, or **'how would you cope with failing to get a position in this program'**.

In each instance, the expectation is the same, and even though it is a crude test of your ability to handle untoward outcome, it is still a common question on the interview train.

Worksheet

♣ 6. How come that you have great letters of recommendation?

Insight

Even though applicants sometimes find this question awkward to answer, it is a fair question to ask, and many times the interviewer is giving the applicant an opportunity to cover multiple grounds in the course of answering one question. As you consider the question more closely, you will discover that there are many parts to it. Not only does it offer you an opportunity to talk about the work experience that enabled you to obtain such excellent letters, it gives you a ground to talk about yourself in an indirect way. Beyond that, you may even use the opportunity to talk about one of the letter writers, as in the case of being a mentor, and how it has influenced your decision to apply to a particular program or follow a particular career path.

For a start, it may be the first time you are hearing such a comment from an interviewer, in which case you are viewed as a desirable applicant. It also makes your work easier, and on your part, the least you can do is not to falter during the interview process.

One point that should not be overlooked as you prepare a response to this question is the fact that great letters of recommendation are never accidental. It is the evidence of the effort on your part in attaining a level of excellence in the course of your work that such letters are written on your behalf. It also means that in addition to performing excellently in the course of doing your work, you have managed to build a sound relationship with your superiors such that they vested in your career success. It is therefore important not only to have a suitable response to this question, but to do all that you can in your capacity to be placed in a position that such a question comes your way.

Answer

It is reassuring to hear that from you.

One of the letters was written by my mentor, Dr. Obinna, a pathologist that I had understudied since I became aware of the field of pathology and its role in the overall practice of medicine. In one of my earlier conversations with him, he acknowledged my early commitment to the field and recognized my ability and predisposition to become a great pathologist. It has been a real privilege to have such a role model.

The second letter was written by the chief of pathology at my medical school in Nigeria. I also connected with her very early in my career journey, and had the opportunity to serve as a research assistant on a study on the subject of cerebral malaria and its histological manifestation. I believe she was impressed with my overall attitude to work, my innate tendency to be optimistic, and the way I relate with my peers and superiors.

Dr. Shaka wrote my third letter. He is a junior lecturer at my medical school and had served as a role model and as someone much younger and had nudged to keep up the good work during my career journey.

I am indebted to all of them, and I am sure they will be very delighted if I should match into UCH Pathology.

Notes

This question offers you one good opportunity to talk about others without been asked to do so. It also allows you to use your association with them to further your course in securing a choice training position. It's another example of 'healthy name-dropping', in the context of an interview process. While one is not sure if you will ever be able to offer a comprehensive response in the example above, it is worthwhile to use the opportunity to talk about one of them, as well as tell about why you are a worthy applicant.

'acknowledgement', is a reasonable start as you respond to the question. Not only do you get to show respect for the interviewer's observation, it is a good basis to start the conversation, rather than start talking about yourself and others.

'healthy name-dropping', as discussed in the preceding paragraphs is right in this instance, enabling you to reiterate the names of those who wrote your letters, but to register the impact they have had on your journey so far and future plans.

'UCH Pathology', is an example of specificity, as it relates to the way to proceed with the conversation, and as highlighted in other sections of this book. While it is not that critical, it is an opportunity to connect with the interviewer on the subject of 'brand', as it relates to the program you are applying to get into. As I mentioned earlier, it is an effort on your part to personalize the conversation to let the interviewer know you are particularly interested in that program.

Key Points

The essentials relating to this question has been fleshed out in the early part of this discussion.

This question is also a reminder to put your effort into doing the best work you can, and to continue on building relationships that are likely to yield the kind of excellent letters of recommendation that are the subject of this conversation.

Lastly, variants of this question may include, **'tell me about Dr. X, I noticed that she is one of your letter writers'**, **'what works did you do to get such great LORs'**, or **'tell me about your experience with Dr. X'**.

As you can see, the intention of the interview is the same, all in an effort to gain a better understanding of what was written about you.

Worksheet

♣ 7. What is your picture of an ideal resident?

Insight

This one of those hypothetical questions that makes one wonder what exactly does the interviewer want, beyond the formality of an interview exercise. Since this question is about the ideal resident, and knowing fully well that such individuals are such a rarity, all that one can do is to respond to the question in an hypothetical sense.

Having said that, there are tiny windows of opportunity to shine as an applicant in the way one chooses to address the question. In my experience working with residency applicant, my general advice is to avoiding walking into a trap by trying to describe yourself as anything close to one. If anything, you are likely to be viewed in a good light to acknowledge the fact that, as an applicant you personally don't quite fit such a description, but that it is an aspiration you plan to continue to strive for.

In line with the comments made in the earlier paragraphs, one is left with no option but to go through the list of the top attributes sought after in every resident. Having considered different approaches to tackling the question, my favorite formula is one that combines the academic, personality, and behavioral attributes. Such an all-encompassing take on the question leaves the interviewer with the task of what exactly they plan to extract from such an elaborate response.

Answer

For a start, I hope you know my response to this question is in no way a description of me of an applicant.

Personally, as a work in progress, it is an ideal that I continue to strive for. Rather than provide you an extensive list of the attributes of the ideal resident, I will like to start with the attributes that I possess, and if time permits tell you about the other desirable qualities, some of which I am yet to achieve.

Respect of the individual comes on top of my list, as it applies to patients, colleagues and my superiors. Rather than focus on academic ability of the resident, an asset that I believe is common to most residents, the attitude to work rides high among the qualities that I consider important as a resident. Using the corollary of the 'cheerful giver', there is nothing as pleasing as observing a 'cheerful resident' who is dedicated to the care of patients, as well as to having an excellent relationship with all that are involved in the attainment of this common goal. Third on my list, is the sense of compassion; this particular trait, while it is talked about by many, is not always evident in our interaction with one another. This particular quality addresses the issues of selfishness and insensitivity that is often observed in our day to day interactions.

The other attributes that I consider desirable and I would expect in an ideal resident include patience, self-confidence, and the ability to better handle stress in the course of my work as a resident. These attributes, I believe are important, and remain one of my priorities as I begin this journey.

Notes

It is important to note that there are many ways to address this particular question, and as such, you should take the time to craft a response that works best for you.

One other observation worth noting is the fact that, the list of qualities that describe an ideal resident is extensive, and it will be a waste of time on your part, as well as on the part of the interviewer that devote the period of the conversation to talking about hypothetical qualities that barely pertain to you, the applicant.

A closer look at the pattern will also reveal the fact that in a way, you have managed to reiterate some of your strengths, and touch on some of your weaknesses. This particular presentation is an excellent demonstration of how to make an optimum use of an hypothetical question to further your case as an applicant during an interview.

'disclaimer', a good tactic in choosing not to compare yourself to the so-called, 'ideal resident'. Anything short of such an attitude may not be received in good taste by the interviewer. It is also a demonstration of 'enlightened humility', one of the critical attributes that every resident should possess.

'the list of three', is another useful tactic where you intentionally limit the stated number of attributes to two, or at most three among the ones that you identify with, and the same number for the other attributes of an ideal resident that you aspire to attain.

'closure', is key if you want to get the most out of this question. There is no point going through the exercise without finding one way or the other to identify with one or two of the attributes that you have identified.

Key Points

On the surface, this question seems inconsequential in the scheme of things in its relevance to the applicant during an interview session, but as you would have noticed, a thoughtful dissection of the subject revealed that it is not a bad question to be presented with after all. Like every event in life, it all depends on how one chooses to handle it.

Again, as it has been reiterated on other pages of this book, doing justice to this question boils down to systematic preparation. Using your worksheet, or a separate notepad, draw up your style of approach to this particular question and put it to test.

Other variants of this question may include, **'which resident is your ideal role model?'**, or **'who is a perfect resident?'**.

Worksheet

♣ 8. What are your interests outside of medicine?

Insight

This question is a rather common one, offering an interviewee a soft landing, and serving as a starting point during an interview session. Often, this question is encountered halfway through or toward the end of an interview session. The timing of the question is however not as important as what the applicant choose to make of the question. Rather than read any meaning to the sequence of the question, it is better to treat the question with the same level of seriousness that one would accord the most anticipated question during an interview exercise.

In itself, it is a nice question to be presented with, especially if one has had the time to practice and rehearse for an optimal response. It is important to pay attention to the salient feature of the question, especially the word, 'interests'. While the word may pass for your hobbies, it is important to be sure what exactly the interviewer expects of you. Some have construed the question to mean a medical subspecialty of interest, and have responded to the question as such. Others have equated it to mean hobbies, especially athletic and sporting activities, while others have interpreted it to mean voluntary activities in service to the community. Unless there are specific instructions from the interviewer, to go in a particular direction, the option is left to applicants to address the question along a line that they are most comfortable with. Some choose a mix of interests that covers sports, community service, and leisurely activities, while others stick to one specific group.

Once clarity is established about the intention of the interviewer, one is faced with the question of how many interests one is allowed to reference in the course of answering such a question. In my practice of guiding applicants through this exercise, I generally advise using the 'list of three', but to start with the most significant of the three. In other words, if your main interest is swimming, but you also do hiking and long distance running, you may want to dwell more on your swimming exploits. As you probably know at this point in reading this book, you are expected to do more than listing these interests, but to find opportunities, if possible to connect your engagement in such activities with how it offers you some benefit or the other.

Answer

Over the years, I have developed a number of interests outside of my usual work routine. Not only do I enjoy hiking and long-distance running, swimming however is my favorite recreational activity.

In my freshman year of high school, I joined the junior swimming team, and since then I have never stopped. Even though I don't engage in the sport at a competitive level, twice a week and at least once over the weekend, I make sure that I visit the local swimming club to do a few laps. It surely has kept me in good shape and enabled me to maintain a decent stamina. Apart from usual benefits of regularly engaging in swimming exercises, I use the opportunity to connect with individuals outside of the hospital setting. I highly recommend it as a form of aerobic exercise suitable for all ages.

With respect to long distance running, the hectic study routine at medical school meant I could only engage in it will all seriousness during vacations. As you know, the traffic in the city does not help my trying to run on local roads.

Hiking is my least favorite leisurely activity. I have not participated in hiking for some months now. I don't quite know when I will get back to it, but I would rather trade it in for swimming. It is also more of hassle to travel to suitable geographical locations to engage in such activities.

Notes

One observation that is evident in the way that I chose to tackle this question is the fact that my answer, the 'list of three', were limited to athletic activities. Though, it was intentional on my part, it is a demonstration of how it is possible to take this question in different directions, unless the interviewer prefers a specific direction.

'the list of three', is already explained as a convenient tactic suitable in this instance. The limitation of the approach is the constraint on time, and in many instances one may not be able to go past the first item on the list.

'clarification', may be necessary where the intention of the interviewer in not clear-cut. The last thing you want to end up doing is to spent the time talking about bird watching when you are expected to talk about a particular aspect of medicine.

'engagement', is key if you want to get the most out of this question. On rare occasions, I have heard applicants share their excitement when were able to connect with the interviewer over a shared interest.

Key Points

The essential points in dealing with this question center on the issue of clarity as to what the interviewer expects of the applicant.

The much talked variants of this question include **'tell me about your hobbies', 'what do you do during your spare time?', or 'what else do you do when you are not working?'**

Worksheet

♣ 9. Talking about leadership roles, what experience comes to mind and how did it go?

Insight

This particular question features from time to time, although it is not as popular as the questions addressed so far in this book. It is also one of the very direct questions one can expect during an interview, and one that is often well rehearsed by many.

The issue with this question according some applicant is what to do if their record of a leadership role is not as robust as one would expect. In dealing with this concern, my take on the issue is that the question is less interested in the magnitude of the role, as in having a nice title, as it is about you're your role entailed and what impact you had during a moment in time. Playing a leadership role could be in the setting of a medical outreach team, a research study group, or as part of a patient advocacy group. Even for those who think they possess little in the way of leadership experience, they are often surprised once the process of combing through their resume reveal areas in the course of their career where they have played such roles.

As this question taps into an event that the applicant was once involved or still involved in, the whole exercise of delivering a suitable response becomes a recount of the overall experience, including the favorable and unfavorable aspects. Rather than let the clock run on with you devoting all the time talking about the experience, it is important to plot the whole conversation in such a way that the reference activity, your role as a leader, and lessons gained from the experience are all conveyed in a meaningful way to the interviewer.

Answer

It is not often that I get to play a leadership role in the course of my study or brief experience of work. In general, I am a silent worker who prefers to get the job done and strive to make all those involved in a task look good.

One activity that readily comes to mind is my current role as a lead researcher in a small-size research forum, overseeing a group of six contributors. My primary role is essentially administrative in nature, and include synchronizing of participant's calendars for group meetings, setting up timelines for various milestones, ensuring fair allocation of work roles to participants, and meeting regularly with the hospital's statistician.

The experience itself has been interesting, although is challenging at times. In playing this role, I get to learn a lot more about members of the group than I would ordinarily have. To fully play this role, I have had to brush up on my statistical analysis skills, work on my ability to multitask, and be adept at time management. It has not been easy overall, and I have had to be creative to achieve a manageable balance between playing the role, and to fully engage in my studies as a final year medical student.

Looking back, I am glad I chose to work with the group, and to be nominated for the role of leadership. It has definitely taken me out of my comfort zone, and has motivated me to interact more with all the individuals that are involved in the project.

I will definitely do it again.

Notes

While this question appears to be straight forward, the response to the question needs to be engaging, and be delivered in such a way that the interviewer can almost feel your joy of playing the role, as well as your frustration, if any. Try to make the subject interesting as it is the kind of conversation that has the potential to roll on to other subjects.

Among the unique features of the answer render in response to this question are the following:

'**subject matter**, should be selected such that you have the opportunity to talk about an element of your resume that the interview may not touch on due to time constraints. In this particular case, the involvement of the applicant in research is an excellent option.

'**being real'**, is equally important, especially as one narrates the experience. It is perfectly okay to be open, and let the interview know about the ups and down, as well as what you have learned through the experience.

'**closing'**, is key in the ending part of the conversation, and should be designed to reveal your overall enthusiasm for the task, including the likelihood of taking up such a role when you become one of the residents in their program.

Key Points

Overall, this is a fair question, one that offers both the interviewer and the applicant a reasonable opportunity to have an engaging conversation.

With respect to having variants of this question, there are only so many ways that this question may be dressed in order not to make it monotonous. Such variants include **'what leadership role did you engage in lately?'**, **'what are your thoughts with taking up a leadership role as one of our residents?'**, or **"tell me about your experience of leadership in the community outreach team that you referenced in your resume'**.

In all the cases, you should be prepared to talk about the nature of the activity, your role as a member and a leader in the group, and the skills you have gained from the experience.

Worksheet

♣ 10. What factors will influence how you will rank a program during the Match?

Insight

This question is not one of those questions that the applicant likes to address, especially early in the course of the interview season.

One reason is the fact that it is often construed as misleading, and may give the false impression that the applicant is a much sought after candidate, especially if the individual in question has a great profile – good scores, favorable year of graduation, as well as an impressive set of letters of recommendation.

On the hand, presenting such a question to an applicant with less desirable profile - one or more attempts in a qualifying examination, unfavorable year of graduation, or a gap since graduation form medical school – may result in an awkward situation where such an applicant finds the question insensitive. Often, the question is randomly selected by the interviewer, and the selection profile may not have been well reviewed to decide if the question is a fair one to present to the applicant.

As an applicant, irrespective of your profile, be it good or suboptimal, it is reasonable to prepare for this question. Rather than consider the question awkward, consider it an opportunity to present yourself as worthy of matching into the program, and do not appear surprised by the question.

For all you know, all the interviewer wants to know is how interested you are in their training program. You will therefore be doing yourself an injustice if you shy away from responding to the question for what it is.

Answer

I know it is quite early in the interview season to begin the talk about ranking, but I am glad that you brought this up early instead of waiting till later in the season or closer to when the selection process takes place.

Since you posed this question, I would like you to know that your training program will be at the top of my rank order list. I am not saying this to impress you, or because I want to make you feel good about me, but one major factor in my decision is that I live in the next town over, less than 30 minutes by car, and even shorter if I choose to hop on the train. Not only is your Pediatric program highly respected, because of my interest in neonatal aspect of pediatrics, there is no better place for me to undergo my residency training.

Notes

In responding to this question, the applicant sometimes feel like it is a trap. Even if one does not plan to rank the program high, it will be inappropriate to make that known that early in the interview season. An alternative take on this question is to avoid offering a response altogether, and emphatically state that you would rather wait till later to confront that issue. To avoid making a mess of the interview experience, a degree of tact is required in the way an applicant answers the question.

In the example shared in this text, one gets a sense that the interviewee was sincere and demonstrated a reasonable degree of authenticity. Many experienced interviewers can see through a pretentious response, and it may be reasonable to stay on the side of indecision, especially if you are unsure of how you feel about the program, and you have other interviews to attend.

In summary, the options available to the applicant include:

'avoidance', is one way to address the question, although most applicants are not adept at doing this in such a way that it does not give a bad impression.

'indecision', is another option, if you can craft a suitable response.

'play', may be the safest option, even if you have other interviews to attend and would rather not take the first two routes to address the question.

Key Points

While this question demands a direct answer, you have an opportunity to express your genuine interest in the program. The fact that you are unable to emphatically state that you will rank the program high does not always mean that you will be penalized, especially if you have good reasons, such as other interviews to attend, spousal or other family considerations. The final decision on the best way to respond to such a question lies with the applicant, and will depend on many factors, some of which may be personal.

While the variants of this particular question are limited, do not make you response a simple 'yes', if you plan to rank the program high, or an ordinary 'no' if you plan to do otherwise. Use the opportunity to express how desirable the program is, how you would like to be one of their residents, and do not let the conversation end on a bland note.

Worksheet

** Remember to get Vol. 2 of this book series.**

♣ Workbook

·

ABOUT THE AUTHOR

Olarewaju Oladipo is an author (fiction and non-fiction) whose writing career began while practicing as an orthopedic surgeon. Following the release of his earlier books "The White Coat" (2006) and "House Calls" (2007), he dedicated the next few years to crafting motivational quotes written using the Twitter handle @3SqMeals as Dr. O' and publishing related books.

Using the experience of the challenges that he encountered at different stages of his medical career, through an organization named KAINJI, he channeled his energy into mentoring young international medical graduates in pursuit of advanced education in the Europe and North America. This work further solidified his engagement in personal development, professional coaching, and counseling.

His works of fiction include the "North Main Street" (mystery) series and the "Once A Doc" (medical fiction) series, with the release of Barber's Haven (2015), 'A Patient called Emma' (2015) and 'Ghost Bus (2016).

'The Sculpture Garden' series is based on actual sculptures and part of an ongoing effort to support the work of local artists in Nigeria. Two Blind Men (2017) was the first of a collection of short stories of the 'Sculpture Garden' series. Tortoise of Many Colors (2017), The Tree of Wonder (2017), and Esther (2018) are other books in the series.

All books are available in paperbacks and eBook at various retail outlets.

Made in United States
Orlando, FL
10 November 2022

24392897R00043